CW01379141

KETO SLOW COOKER COOKBOOK

The Ultimate Ketogenic Diet Guide. Delicious, Easy and Quick Low Carb Recipes for Rapid Weight loss. Improve and Optimize your Life.

Table of Contents

KETO SLOW COOKER COOKBOOK — 1

The Ultimate Ketogenic Diet Guide. Delicious, Easy and Quick Low Carb Recipes for Rapid Weight loss. Improve and Optimize your Life. — 1

- New Mexico Carne Adovada — 11
- Smoky Pork with Cabbage — 13
- Simple Roasted Pork Shoulder — 15
- Flavors Pork Chops — 17
- Tasty Pork Tacos — 19
- Lime Pork Chops — 21
- Chili Pulled Pork — 23
- Ranch Pork Chops — 26
- Onion Pork Chops — 28
- Mahi-Mahi Taco Wraps — 31
- Shrimp Scampi — 33
- Shrimp Tacos — 36
- Fish Curry — 38
- Salmon with Creamy Lemon Sauce — 41
- Salmon with Lemon-Caper Sauce — 45
- Spicy Barbecue Shrimp — 47
- Lemon Dill Halibut — 50
- Coconut Cilantro Curry Shrimp — 52
- Shrimp in Marinara Sauce — 55
- Garlic Shrimp — 58
- Salmon Poached in White Wine and Lemon — 60
- Lemon Pepper Tilapia — 62
- Poached Salmon in Court-Bouillon Recipe — 64

- Braised Squid with Tomatoes and Fennel — 66
- Seafood Stir-Fry Soup — 69
- Shrimp Fajita Soup — 72
- Fish and Tomatoes — 73

Vegetables — 75

- Parmesan Mushrooms — 75
- Mashed Garlic Cauliflower — 77
- Braised Cabbage — 79
- Homemade Vegetable Stock — 83
- Vegetable Korma — 85
- Stuffed Eggplant — 88
- Bacon Cheddar Broccoli Salad — 91
- Cracked-Out Keto Slaw — 94
- Zucchini Pasta — 96
- Twice Baked Spaghetti Squash — 99
- Mushroom Risotto — 102
- Vegan Bibimbap — 104
- Avocado Pesto Kelp Noodles — 107
- Creamy Curry Sauce Noodle Bowl — 109

© Copyright 2020 by Master Kitchen American - All rights reserved.

The following Book is reproduced below with the goal of providing information that is as accurate and reliable as possible. Regardless, purchasing this Book can be seen as consent to the fact that both the publisher and the author of this book are in no way experts on the topics discussed within and that any recommendations or suggestions that are made herein are for entertainment purposes only. Professionals should be consulted as needed prior to undertaking any of the action endorsed herein.

This declaration is deemed fair and valid by both the American Bar Association and the Committee of Publishers Association and is legally binding throughout the United States.

Furthermore, the transmission, duplication, or reproduction of any of the following work including specific information will be considered an illegal act irrespective of if it is done electronically or in print. This extends to creating a secondary or tertiary copy of the work or a recorded copy and is only allowed with the express written consent from the Publisher. All additional right reserved.

The information in the following pages is broadly considered a truthful and accurate account of facts and as such, any inattention, use, or misuse of the information in question by the reader will render any resulting actions solely under their purview. There are no scenarios in which the publisher or the original author of this work can be in any fashion deemed liable for any hardship or damages that may befall them after undertaking information described herein.

Additionally, the information in the following pages is intended only for informational purposes and should thus be thought of as universal. As befitting its nature, it is presented without assurance regarding its prolonged validity or interim quality. Trademarks that are mentioned are done without written consent and can in no way be considered an endorsement from the trademark holder.

New Mexico Carne Adovada

Preparation Time: 30 minutes

Cooking Time: 6 hours

Servings: 4

Ingredients:

2 tsp apple cider vinegar

1 tsp kosher salt

1 tsp ground coriander

1 tsp ground cumin

2 tsp dried Mexican oregano

6 garlic, sliced

1 onion, sliced

2 cups chicken stock

6 -8 ounces dried chilies, rinsed

3 pounds pork shoulder, cubes

Directions:

Put all the items in a pot, except the pork. Simmer it within 30-60 minutes, low.

Remove, then cooldown it within a few minutes.

Puree the batter in batches using a blender.

Put now the pork meat in a baking dish, covering it with the sauce. Chill within 1 to 2 days to marinate, stirring frequently.

Cook it in a slow cooker within 4 to 6 hours, low.

Serve warm.

Nutrition:

Calories 120.2

Fat 5.3g

Carb 11.3g

Protein 8.0g

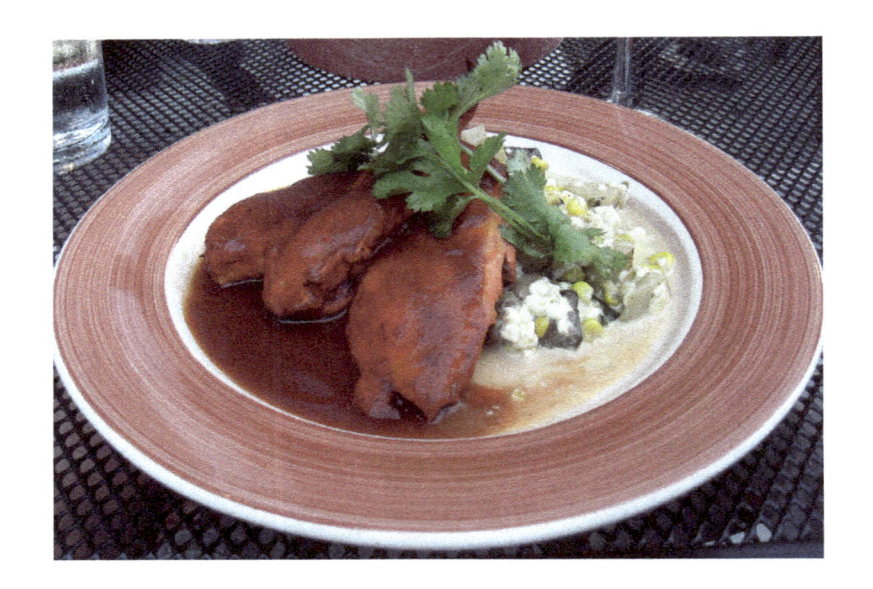

Smoky Pork with Cabbage

Preparation Time: 10 minutes

Cooking Time: 8 hours

Servings: 6

Ingredients:

lbs pastured pork roast

1/3 cup liquid smoke

1/2 cabbage head, chopped

1 cup water

1 tbsp kosher salt

Directions:

Rub pork with kosher salt and place into the slow cooker.

Pour liquid smoke over the pork. Add water.

Cover slow cooker with lid and cook on low for 7 hours.

Remove pork from slow cooker and add cabbage in the bottom of slow cooker.

Now place pork on top of the cabbage.

Cover again and cook for 1 hour more.

Shred pork with a fork and serves.

Nutrition:

Calories 484

Fat 21.5 g

Carbohydrates 3.5 g

Sugar 1.9 g

Protein 65.4 g

Cholesterol 195 mg

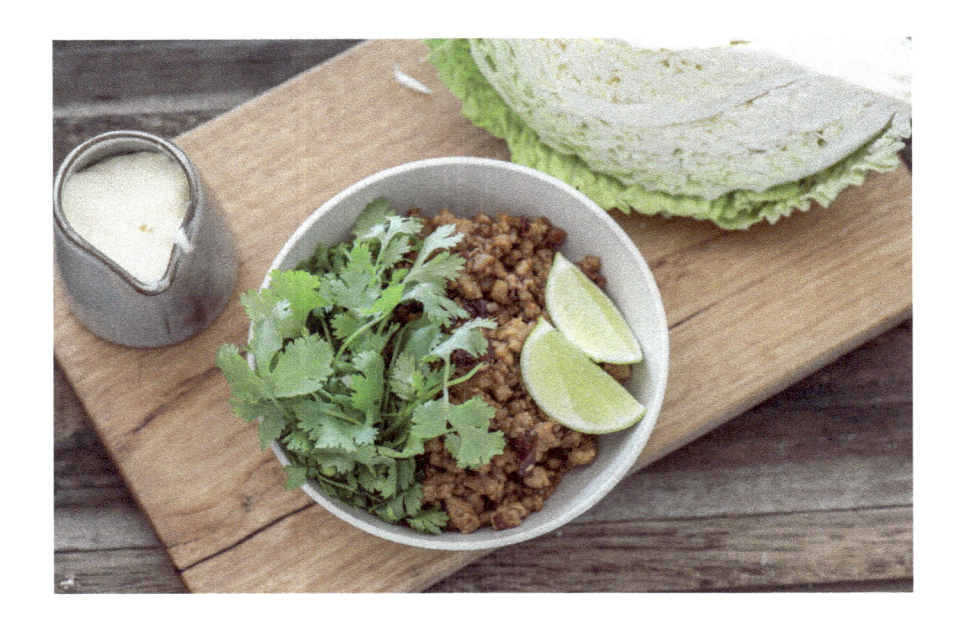

Simple Roasted Pork Shoulder

Preparation Time: 10 minutes

Cooking Time: 9 hours

Servings: 8

Ingredients:

lbs pork shoulder

1 tsp garlic powder

1/2 cup water

1/2 tsp black pepper

1/2 tsp sea salt

Directions:

Season pork with garlic powder, pepper, and salt and place in slow cooker. Add water.

Cover slow cooker with lid and cook on high for 1 hour then turn heat to low and cook for 8 hours.

Remove meat from slow cooker and shred using a fork.

Serve and enjoy.

Nutrition:

Calories 664

Fat 48.5 g

Carbohydrates 0.3 g

Sugar 0.1 g

Protein 52.9 g

Cholesterol 204 mg

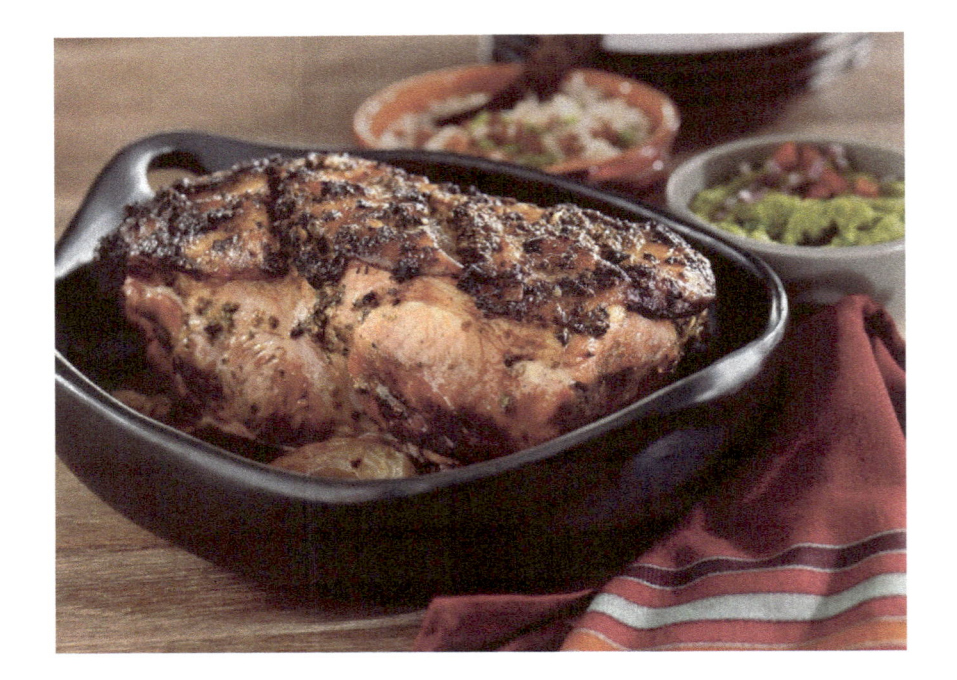

Flavors Pork Chops

Preparation Time: 10 minutes

Cooking Time: 4 hours

Servings: 4

Ingredients:

pork chops

2 garlic cloves, minced

1 cup chicken broth

1 tbsp poultry seasoning

1/4 cup olive oil

Pepper and salt

Directions:

In a bowl, whisk together olive oil, poultry seasoning, garlic, broth, pepper, and salt.

Pour olive oil mixture into the slow cooker then place pork chops into the slow cooker.

Cover slow cooker with lid and cook on high for 4 hours.

Serve and enjoy.

Nutrition:

Calories 386

Fat 32.9 g

Carbohydrates 2.9 g

Sugar 0.7 g

Protein 19.7 g

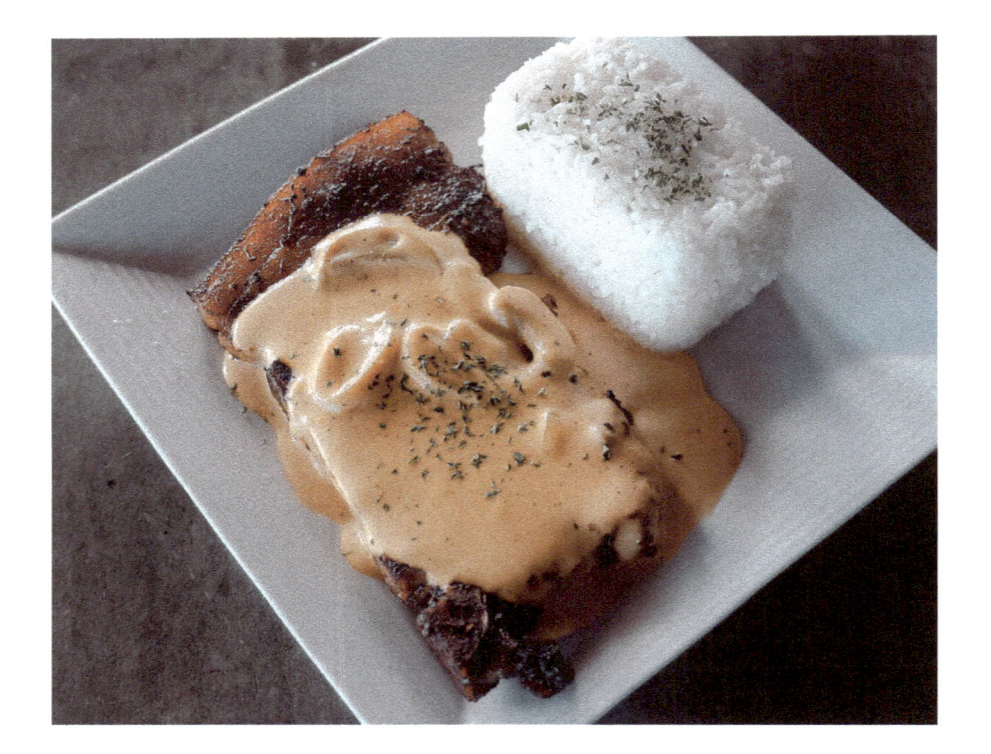

Tasty Pork Tacos

Preparation Time: 15 minutes

Cooking Time: 8 hours

Servings: 8

Ingredients:

2 lbs. pork tenderloin

2 tsp cayenne pepper

24 oz salsa

3 tsp garlic powder

2 tbsp ground cumin

2 tbsp chili powder

1 1/2 tsp salt

Directions:

Place pork tenderloin into the slow cooker.

Mix all rest of the ingredients except salsa in a small bowl.

Rub spice mixture over pork tenderloin. Pour salsa on top of pork tenderloin.

Cook within 8 hours, low. Transfer the pork from slow cooker, and shred using a fork.

Return shredded pork into the slow cooker and stir well with salsa. Serve and enjoy.

Nutrition:

Calories 202

Fat 4.9 g

Carbohydrates 8 g

Sugar 3.1 g

Protein 31.7 g

Cholesterol 83 mg

Fiber 2.4 g

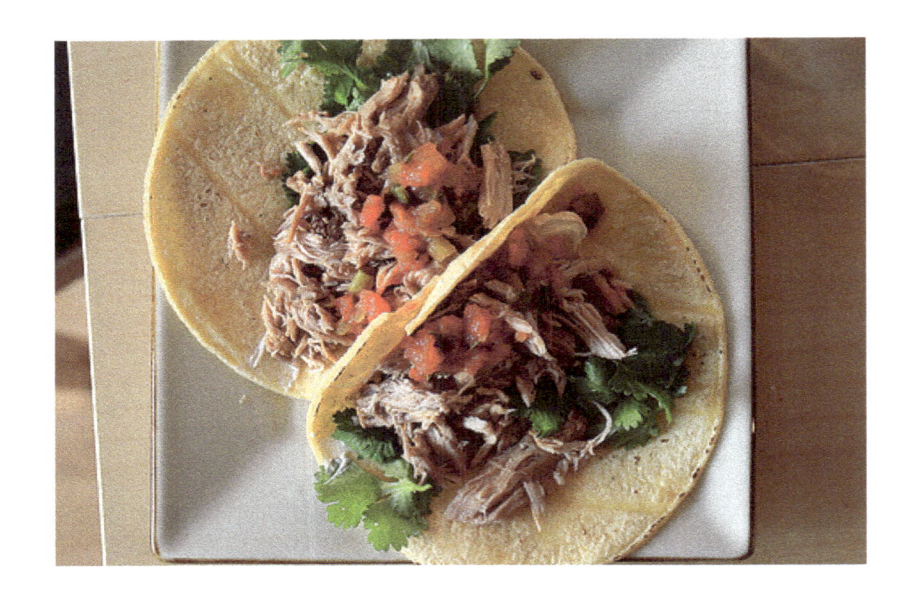

Lime Pork Chops

Preparation Time: 15 minutes

Cooking Time: 4 hours

Servings: 8

Ingredients:

3.32 lb. pork sirloin

¾ teaspoon black pepper

3 tablespoons butter

½ ground cumin

¾ teaspoon salt

½ cup of salsa

¾ teaspoon garlic powder

5 tablespoons lime juice

Directions:

Mix all of the flavorings in a small bowl. Cover the meat all over with the flavoring mixture.

Using a pan, sear the meat in butter over medium-high heat until brown on both sides.

Combine lime juice and salsa in a separate bowl. Mix well.

Put the pork chops inside the slow cooker and pour the salsa mixture on top.

Cook within 3-4 hours, low.

Nutrition:

Calories: 170

Carbs: 8g

Fat: 6g

Protein: 18g

Chili Pulled Pork

Preparation Time: 15 minutes

Cooking Time: 10 hours

Servings: 10

Ingredients:

4 1/2 lb. (2kg) pork butt / shoulder

2 tablespoons chili powder

1 tablespoon salt

1 ½ teaspoon ground cumin

½ teaspoon ground oregano

¼ teaspoon crushed red pepper flakes

Pinch ground cloves

½ cup (120ml) stock or bone broth

1 bay leaf

Directions:

Start by grabbing a bowl and throwing in the chili, salt, cumin, oregano, red pepper flakes, and a pinch of cloves then stir well to combine.

Lay the pork out on a clean plate, remove the skin if applicable, then rub the spice mixture into the pork. Put into the fridge within 1-2 hours.

When you're ready to cook, pop the pork in the bottom of the slow cooker, add the bay leaf and the stock or broth, replace the lid and switch on. Cook on low for 8-10 hours (or overnight) until tender.

Remove the lid, lift the pork from the slow cooker, and place onto a cutting board then shred with two forks.

Serve and enjoy!

Nutrition:

Calories: 210

Carbs: 0g

Fat: 15g

Protein: 0g

© 101 Cooking For Two

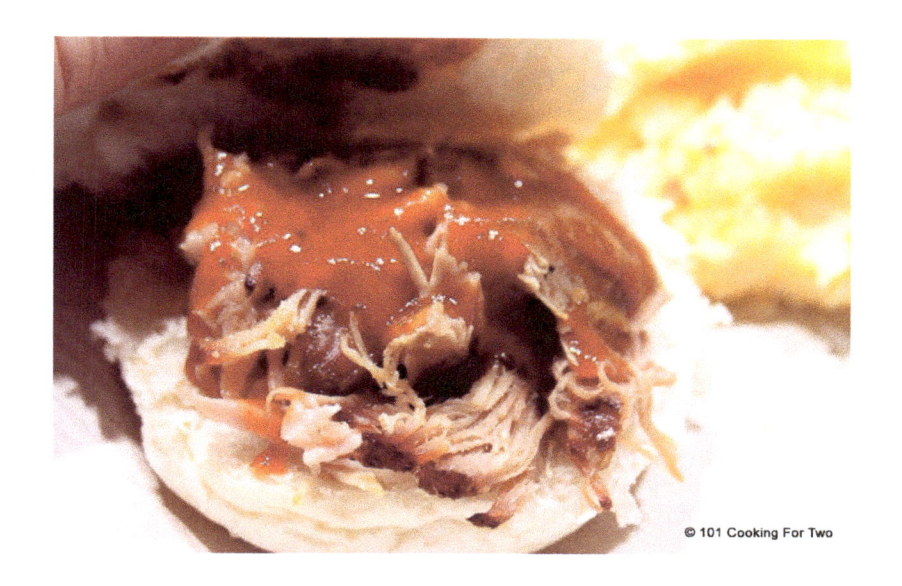

Ranch Pork Chops

Preparation Time: 15 minutes

Cooking Time: 6 hours

Servings: 8

Ingredients:

3 lbs. pork chops

1 tsp garlic powder

1 oz ranch dressing mix

1 oz onion soup mix

22.5 oz cream of mushroom soup

1/2 tsp black pepper

Directions:

Spray slow cooker form inside with cooking spray. Put all listed items into the slow cooker, then mix well. Cook within 6 hours on low. Serve and enjoy.

Nutrition:

Calories 591

Fat 44.6 g

Carbohydrates 5.4 g

Sugar 0.9 g

Protein 39.2 g

Cholesterol 146 mg

Fiber 0.3 g

Net carbs 5.1 g

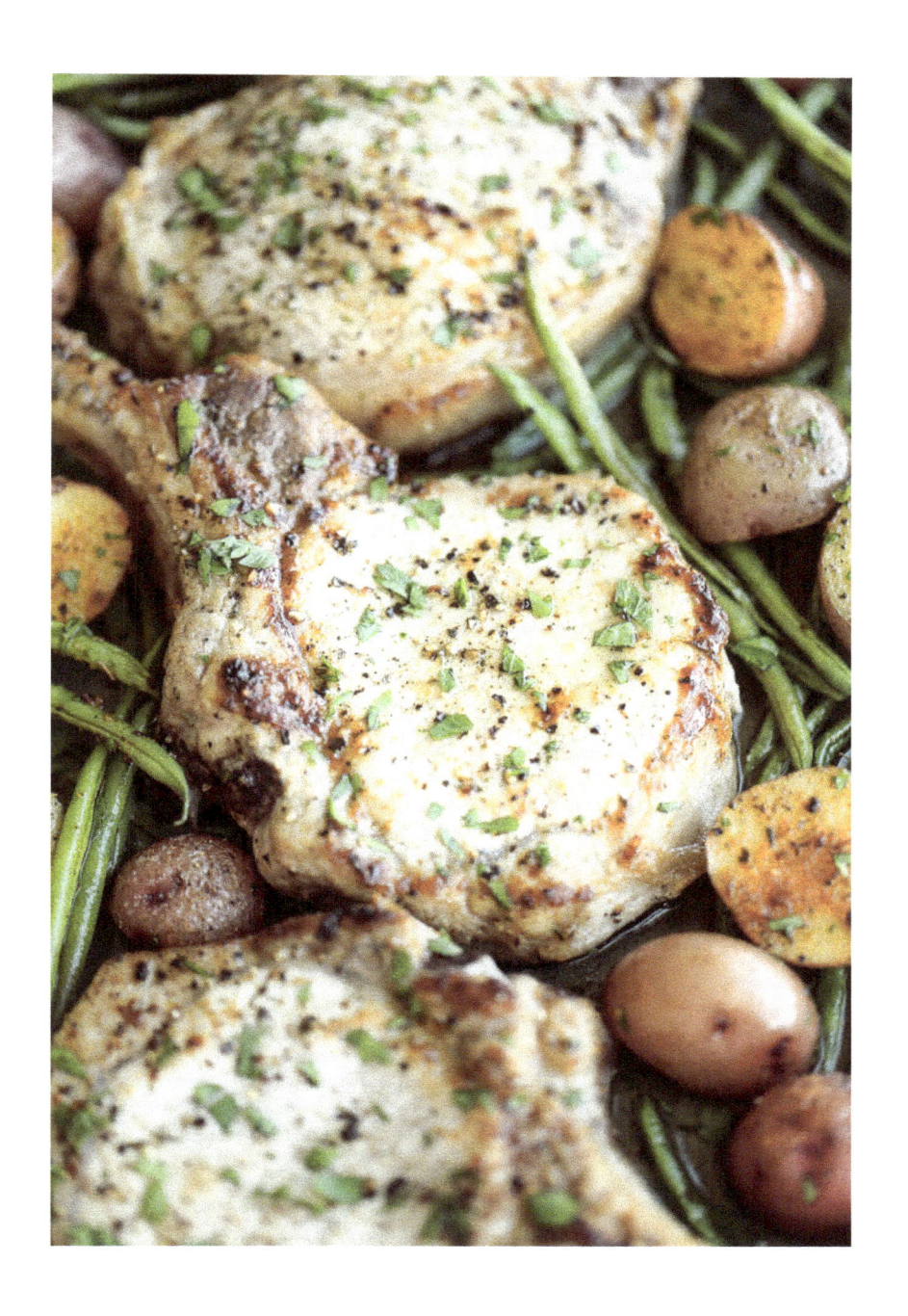

Onion Pork Chops

Preparation Time: 15 minutes

Cooking Time: 6 hours

Servings: 6

Ingredients:

2 lbs. pork chops, boneless

1/4 tsp garlic powder

1 tbsp apple cider vinegar

2 tbsp Worcestershire sauce

1/3 cup butter, sliced

1 large onion, sliced

1/8 tsp red pepper flakes

1 tbsp olive oil

1/4 tsp pepper

1/4 tsp salt

Directions:

Heat-up the olive oil in a pan over medium-high heat. Brown pork chops in hot oil from both sides.

Add remaining ingredients except for onion and butter into the slow cooker and stir well.

Place brown pork chops into the slow cooker and top with butter and onion.

Cook within 6 hours, low. Serve and enjoy.

Nutrition:

Calories 611

Fat 50.2 g

Carbohydrates 3.5 g

Sugar 2.1 g

Protein 34.4 g

Cholesterol 157 mg

Fiber 0.6 g

Net carbs 2.9 g

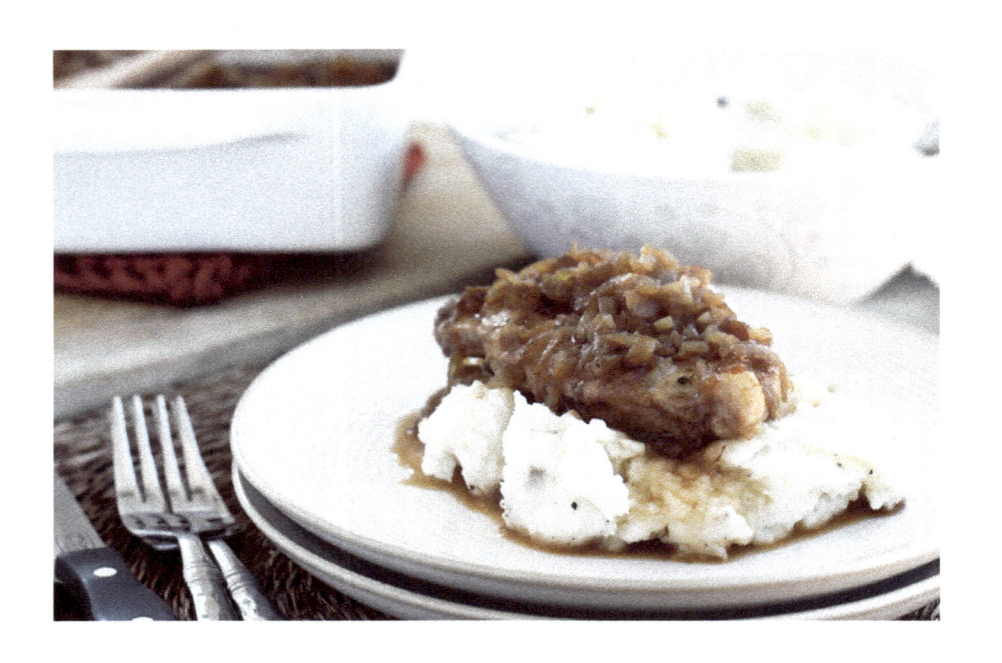

Mahi-Mahi Taco Wraps

Preparation Time: 5 minutes

Cooking Time: 2 hours

Servings: 6

Ingredients:

1-pound Mahi-Mahi, wild-caught

½ cup cherry tomatoes

1 green bell pepper

1/4 medium red onion

½ teaspoon garlic powder

1 teaspoon of sea salt

½ teaspoon ground black pepper

1 teaspoon chipotle pepper

½ teaspoon dried oregano

1 teaspoon cumin

2 tablespoons avocado oil

1/4 cup chicken stock

1 medium avocado, diced

1 cup sour cream

6 large lettuce leaves

Directions:

Grease a 6-quarts slow cooker with oil, place fish in it and then pour in chicken stock.

Stir together garlic powder, salt, black pepper, chipotle pepper, oregano, and cumin and then season fish with half of this mixture.

Layer fish with tomatoes, pepper, and onion, season with remaining spice mixture, and shut with lid.

Plugin the slow cooker, then cook fish for 2 hours at a high heat setting or until cooked.

When done, evenly spoon fish among lettuce, top with avocado and sour cream, and serve.

Nutrition:

Calories: 193.6

Fat: 12g

Protein: 17g

Carbs: 5g

Fiber: 3g

Sugar: 2.5g

Shrimp Scampi

Preparation Time: 5 minutes

Cooking Time: 2 hours & 30 minutes

Servings: 4

Ingredients:

1 pound wild-caught shrimps, peeled & deveined

1 tablespoon minced garlic

1 teaspoon salt

½ teaspoon ground black pepper

1/2 teaspoon red pepper flakes

2 tablespoons chopped parsley

2 tablespoons avocado oil

2 tablespoons unsalted butter

1/2 cup white wine

1 tablespoon lemon juice

1/4 cup chicken broth

½ cup grated parmesan cheese

Directions:

Place all the ingredients except for shrimps and cheese in a 6-quart slow cooker and whisk until combined.

Add shrimps and stir until evenly coated and shut with lid.

Cook in the slow cooker for 1 hour and 30 minutes to 2 hours and 30 minutes at low heat setting or until cooked.

Then top with parmesan cheese and serve.

Nutrition:

Calories: 234

Total Fat: 14.7g

Protein: 23.3g

Carbs: 2.1g

Fiber: 0.1g

Sugar: 2g

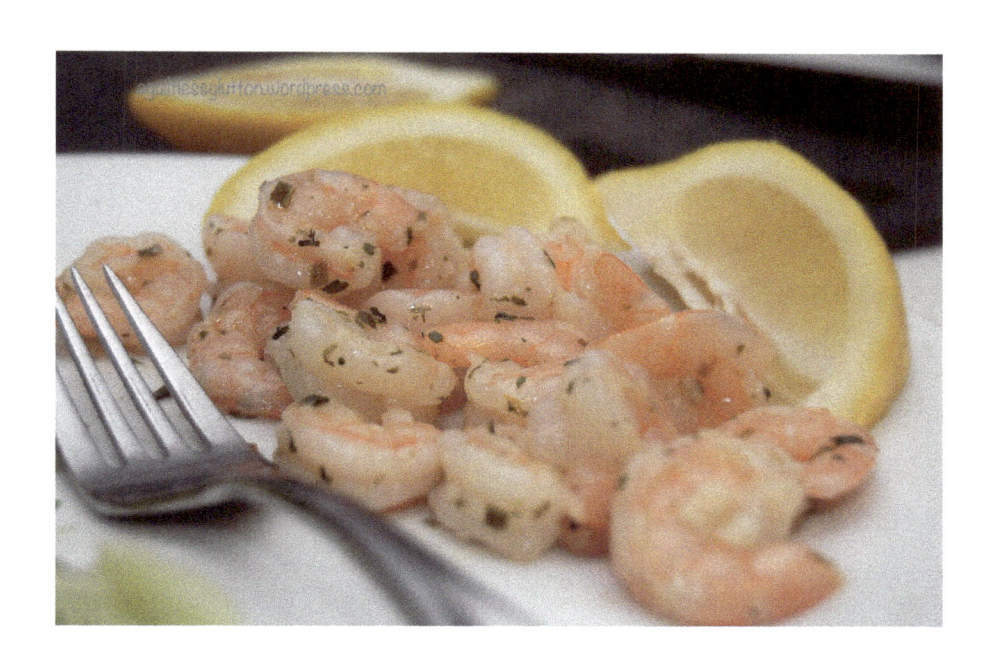

Shrimp Tacos

Preparation Time: 5 minutes

Cooking Time: 3 hours

Servings: 6

Ingredients:

1 pound medium wild-caught shrimp, peeled and tails off

12-ounce fire-roasted tomatoes, diced

1 small green bell pepper, chopped

½ cup chopped white onion

1 teaspoon minced garlic

½ teaspoon of sea salt

½ teaspoon ground black pepper

½ teaspoon red chili powder

½ teaspoon cumin

¼ teaspoon cayenne pepper

2 tablespoons avocado oil

1/2 cup salsa

4 tablespoons chopped cilantro

1 ½ cup sour cream

2 medium avocados, diced

Directions:

Rinse shrimps, layer into a 6-quarts slow cooker, and drizzle with oil.

Add tomatoes, stir until mixed, then add peppers and remaining ingredients except for sour cream and avocado and stir until combined.

Plugin the slow cooker, shut with lid, and cook for 2 to 3 hours at low heat setting or 1 hour and 30 minutes to 2 hours at high heat setting or until shrimps turn pink.

When done, serve shrimps with avocado and sour cream.

Nutrition:

Calories: 369

Fat: 27.5g

Protein: 21.2g

Carbs: 9.2g

Fiber: 5g

Sugar: 5g

Fish Curry

Preparation Time: 5 minutes

Cooking Time: 4 hours 7 30 minutes

Servings: 6

Ingredients:

2.2 pounds wild-caught white fish fillet, cubed

18-ounce spinach leaves

4 tablespoons red curry paste, organic

14-ounce coconut cream, unsweetened and full-fat

14-ounce water

Directions:

Plug in a 6-quart slow cooker and let preheat at high heat setting.

In the meantime, whisk together coconut cream and water until smooth.

Place fish into the slow cooker, spread with curry paste, and then pour in coconut cream mixture.

Cook within 2 hours at a high setting or 4 hours at low heat setting until tender.

Then add spinach and continue cooking for 20 to 30 minutes or until spinach leaves wilt.

Serve straight away.

Nutrition:

Calories: 323

Fat: 51.5g

Protein: 41.3g

Carbs: 7g

Fiber: 2.2g

Sugar: 2.3g

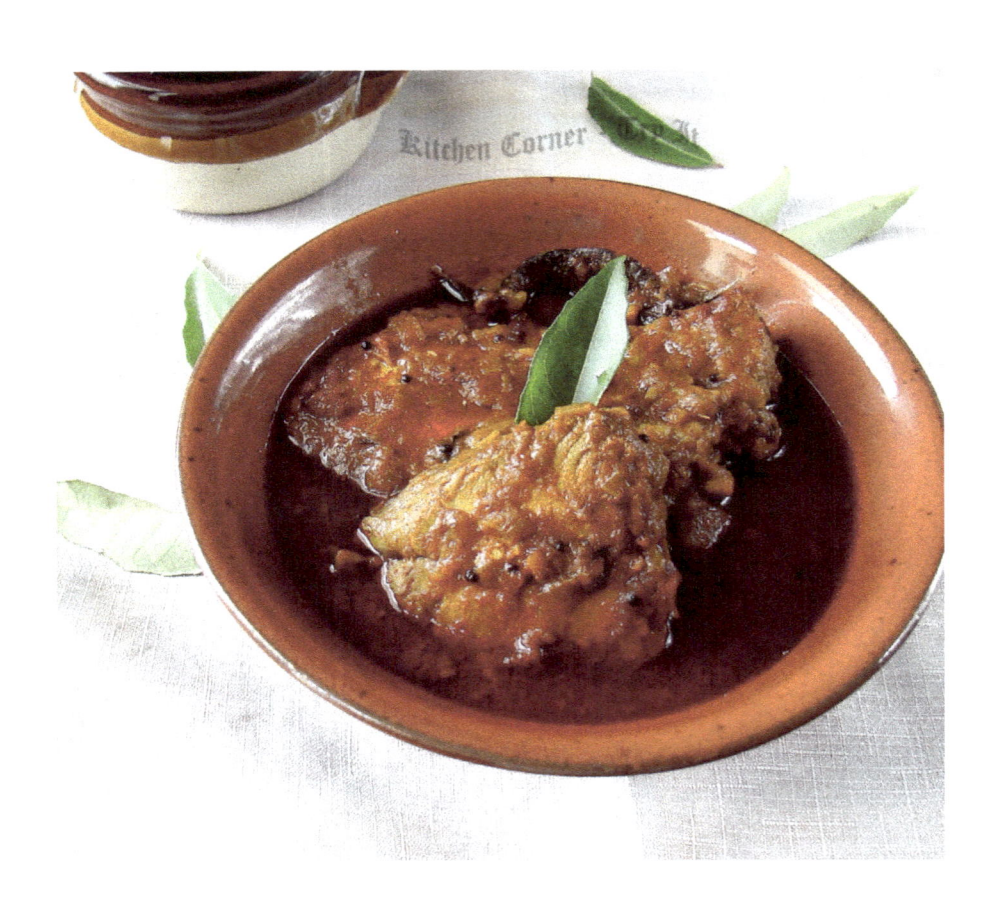

Salmon with Creamy Lemon Sauce

Preparation Time: 5 minutes

Cooking Time: 2 hours & 15 minutes

Servings: 6

Ingredients:

For the Salmon:

2 pounds wild-caught salmon fillet, skin-on

1 teaspoon garlic powder

1 ½ teaspoon salt

1 teaspoon ground black pepper

1/2 teaspoon red chili powder

1 teaspoon Italian Seasoning

1 lemon, sliced

1 lemon, juiced

2 tablespoons avocado oil

1 cup chicken broth

For the Creamy Lemon Sauce:

Chopped parsley, for garnish

1/8 teaspoon lemon zest

1/4 cup heavy cream

1/4 cup grated parmesan cheese

Directions:

Line a 6-quart slow cooker with parchment sheet spread its bottom with lemon slices, top with salmon and drizzle with oil.

Stir together garlic powder, salt, black pepper, red chili powder, Italian seasoning, and oil until combined and rub this mixture all over salmon.

Pour lemon juice and broth around the fish and shut with lid.

Cook in the slow cooker within 2 hours at a low heat setting.

In the meantime, set the oven at 400 degrees F and let preheat.

When fish is done, lift out an inner pot of slow cooker, place into the oven, then cook within 5 to 8 minutes or until the top is nicely browned.

Lift out the fish using a parchment sheet and keep it warm.

Remove, transfer juices to a medium skillet pan, place it over medium-high heat, and then bring to boil and cook for 1 minute.

Turn heat to a low level, whisk the cream into the sauce, and lemon zest and parmesan cheese and cook for 2 to 3 minutes or until thickened.

Cut salmon in pieces, then top each portion with lemon sauce and serve.

Nutrition:

Calories: 340

Fat: 20g

Protein: 32g

Carbs: 8g

Fiber: 2g

Sugar: 2g

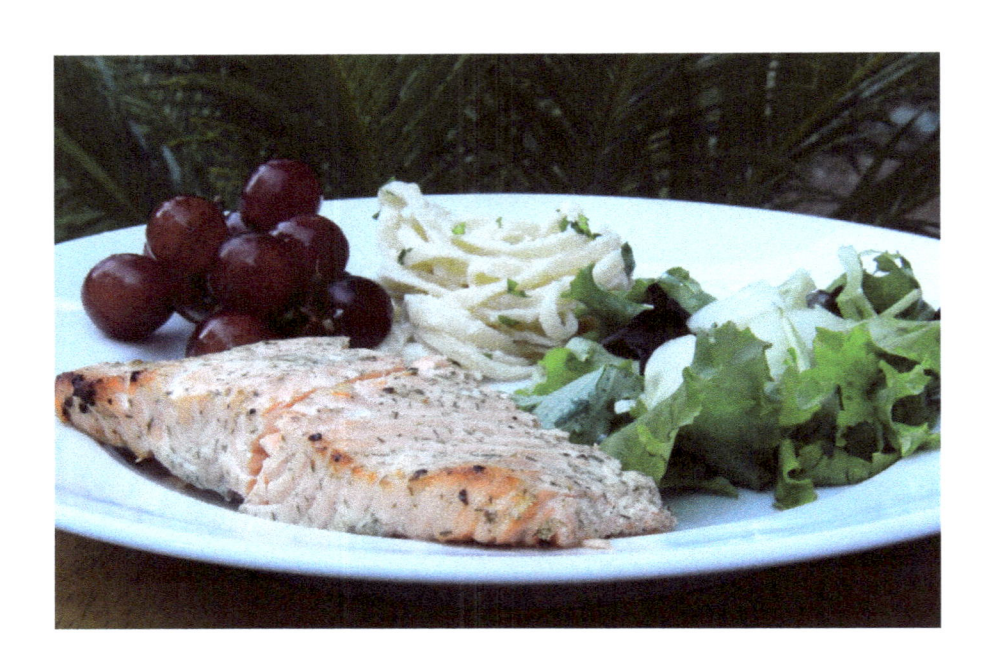

Salmon with Lemon-Caper Sauce

Preparation Time: 5 minutes

Cooking Time: 1 hour & 30 minutes

Servings: 6

Ingredients:

1 pound wild-caught salmon fillet

2 teaspoon capers, rinsed and mashed

1 teaspoon minced garlic

1 teaspoon salt

½ teaspoon ground black pepper

1/2 teaspoon dried oregano

1 teaspoon lemon zest

2 tablespoons lemon juice

4 tablespoons unsalted butter

Directions:

Cut salmon into 4 pieces, then season with salt and black pepper and sprinkle lemon zest on top.

Arrange a 6-quart slow cooker with parchment paper, place seasoned salmon pieces on it, and shut with lid.

Set to cook in the slow cooker within 1 hour and 30 minutes or until salmon is cooked through.

Prepare lemon-caper sauce and for this, place a small saucepan over low heat, add butter and let it melt.

Then add capers, garlic, lemon juice, stir until mixed and simmer for 1 minute.

Remove saucepan from heat and stir in oregano.

When salmon is cooked, spoon lemon-caper sauce on it and serve.

Nutrition:

Calories: 368.5

Fat: 26.6g

Protein: 19.5g

Carbs: 2.7g

Fiber: 0.3g

Sugar: 2g

Spicy Barbecue Shrimp

Preparation Time: 5 minutes

Cooking Time: 1 hour & 30 minutes

Servings: 6

Ingredients:

1 1/2 pounds large wild-caught shrimp, unpeeled

1 green onion, chopped

1 teaspoon minced garlic

1 ½ teaspoon salt

¾ teaspoon ground black pepper

1 teaspoon Cajun seasoning

1 tablespoon hot pepper sauce

¼ cup Worcestershire Sauce

1 lemon, juiced

2 tablespoons avocado oil

1/2 cup unsalted butter, chopped

Directions:

Place all the ingredients except for shrimps in a 6-quart slow cooker and whisk until mixed.

Plugin the slow cooker, then shut with lid and cook for 1 hour and 30 minutes at a high heat setting.

Then take out ½ cup of this sauce and reserve.

Add shrimps to slow cooker.

Nutrition:

Calories: 321

Fat: 21.4g

Protein: 27.3g

Carbs: 4.8g

Fiber: 2.4g

Sugar: 1.2g

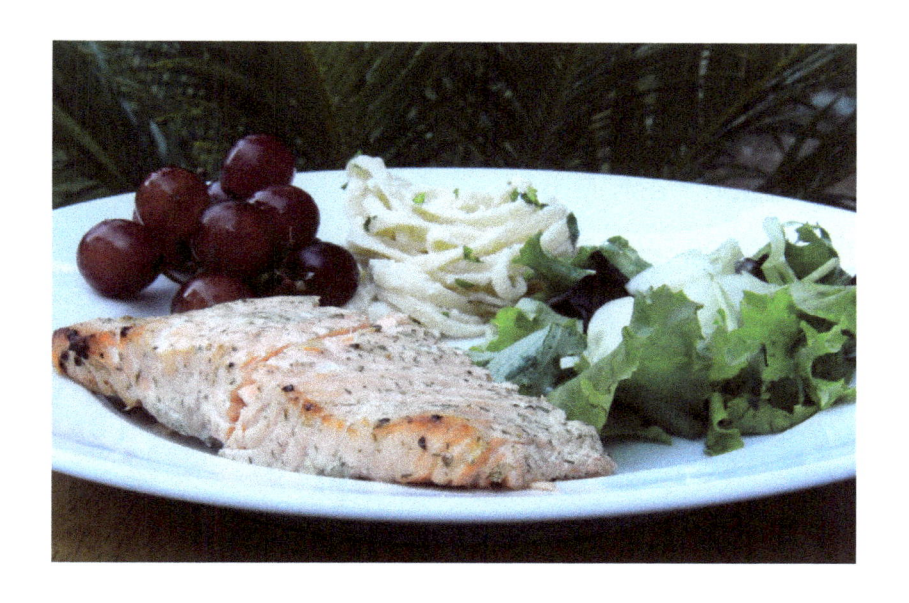

Lemon Dill Halibut

Preparation Time: 15 minutes

Cooking Time: 2 hours

Servings: 2

Ingredients:

12-ounce wild-caught halibut fillet

1 teaspoon salt

½ teaspoon ground black pepper

1 1/2 teaspoon dried dill

1 tablespoon fresh lemon juice

3 tablespoons avocado oil

Directions:

Cut an 18-inch piece of aluminum foil, halibut fillet in the middle, and then season with salt and black pepper.

Whisk the remaining ingredients, drizzle this mixture over halibut, then crimp foil's edges and place it into a 6-quart slow cooker.

Cook within 1 hour and 30 minutes or 2 hours at high heat setting or until cooked.

When done, carefully open the crimped edges and check the fish; it should be tender and flaky.

Serve straight away.

Nutrition:

Calories: 321.5

Fat: 21.4g

Protein: 32.1g

Carbs: 0g

Fiber: 0g

Sugar: 0.6g

Coconut Cilantro Curry Shrimp

Preparation Time: 15 minutes

Cooking Time: 2 hours & 30 minutes

Servings: 4

Ingredients:

1 pound wild-caught shrimp, peeled and deveined

2 ½ teaspoon lemon garlic seasoning

2 tablespoons red curry paste

4 tablespoons chopped cilantro

30 ounces coconut milk, unsweetened

16 ounces of water

Directions:

Whisk together all the ingredients except for shrimps and 2 tablespoons cilantro and add to a 4-quart slow cooker.

Plugin the slow cooker, shut with lid, and cook for 2 hours at high heat setting or 4 hours at low heat setting.

Then add shrimps, toss until evenly coated and cook for 20 to 30 minutes at high heat settings or until shrimps are pink.

Garnish shrimps with remaining cilantro and serve.

Nutrition:

Calories: 160.7

Total Fat: 8.2g

Protein: 19.3g

Carbs: 2.4g

Fiber: 0.5g

Sugar: 1.4g

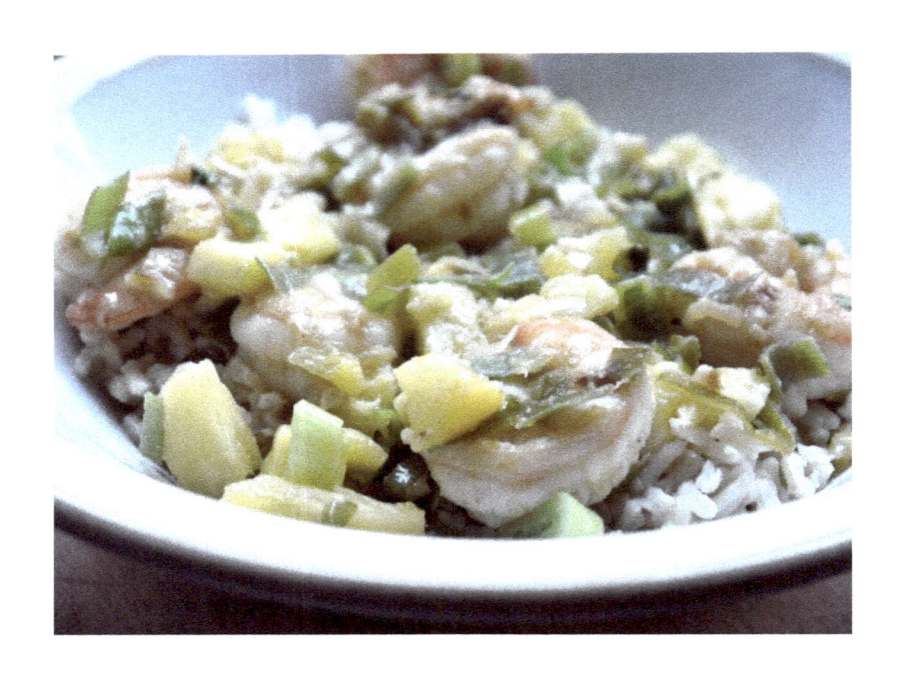

Shrimp in Marinara Sauce

Preparation Time: 15 minutes

Cooking Time: 5 hours & 10 minutes

Servings: 5

Ingredients:

1 pound cooked wild-caught shrimps, peeled and deveined

14.5-ounce crushed tomatoes

½ teaspoon minced garlic

1 teaspoon salt

1/2 teaspoon seasoned salt

¼ teaspoon ground black pepper

½ teaspoon crushed red pepper flakes

1/2 teaspoon dried basil

1/2 teaspoon dried oregano

½ tablespoons avocado oil

6-ounce chicken broth

2 tablespoon minced parsley

1/2 cup grated Parmesan cheese

Directions:

Place all the ingredients except for shrimps, parsley, and cheese in a 4-quart slow cooker and stir well.

Then plug in the slow cooker, shut with lid, and cook for 4 to 5 hours at a low heat setting.

Then add shrimps and parsley, stir until mixed and cook for 10 minutes at high heat setting.

Garnish shrimps with cheese and serve.

Nutrition:

Calories: 358.8

Fat: 25.1g

Protein: 26g

Carbs: 7.2g

Fiber: 1.5g

Sugar: 3.6g

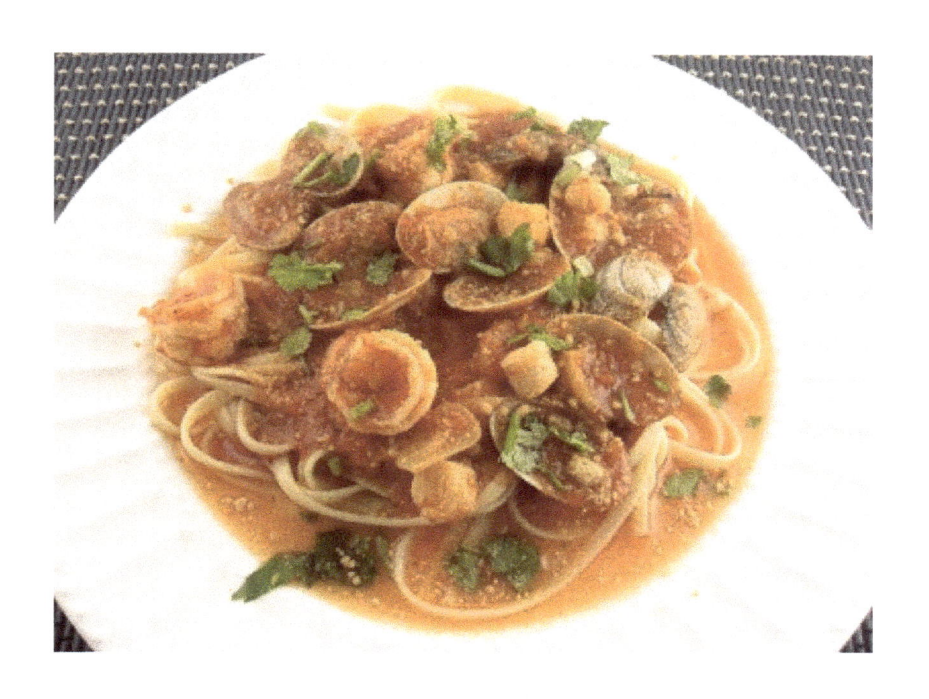

Garlic Shrimp

Preparation Time: 5 minutes

Cooking Time: 1 hour

Servings: 5

Ingredients:

For the Garlic Shrimp:

1 1/2 pounds large wild-caught shrimp, peeled and deveined

1/4 teaspoon ground black pepper

1/8 teaspoon ground cayenne pepper

2 ½ teaspoons minced garlic

1/4 cup avocado oil

4 tablespoons unsalted butter

For the Seasoning:

1 teaspoon onion powder

1 tablespoon garlic powder

1 tablespoon salt

2 teaspoons ground black pepper

1 tablespoon paprika

1 teaspoon cayenne pepper

1 teaspoon dried oregano

1 teaspoon dried thyme

Directions:

Stir together all the ingredients for seasoning, garlic, oil, and butter and add to a 4-quart slow cooker. Plugin the slow cooker, shut with lid, and cook for 25 to 30 minutes at high heat setting or until cooked. Then add shrimps, toss until evenly coated, and continue cooking for 20 to 30 minutes at high heat setting or until shrimps are pink.

When done, transfer shrimps to a serving plate, top with sauce, and serve.

Nutrition:

Calories: 233.6

Fat: 11.7g

Protein: 30.9g

Carbs: 1.2g

Fiber: 0g

Sugar: 0g

Salmon Poached in White Wine and Lemon

Preparation Time: 15 minutes

Cooking Time: 2 hours

Servings: 4

Ingredients:

2 cups of water

1 cup cooking wine, white

1 lemon, sliced thin

1 small mild onion, sliced thin

1 bay leaf

1 mixed bunch fresh tarragon, dill, and parsley

2.2 pounds salmon fillet, skin on

1 teaspoon salt

1 teaspoon ground black pepper

Directions:

Add all fixings, except salmon and seasoning, to the slow cooker. Cover, cook on low for 1 hour.

Season the salmon, place in the slow cooker skin-side down.

Cover, cook on low for another hour. Serve.

Nutrition:

Calories: 216

Carbs: 1g

Fat: 12g

Protein: 23

Lemon Pepper Tilapia

Preparation Time: 5 minutes

Cooking Time: 3 hours

Servings: 6

Ingredients:

6 wild-caught Tilapia fillets

4 teaspoons lemon-pepper seasoning, divided

6 tablespoons unsalted butter, divided

1/2 cup lemon juice, fresh

Directions:

Put each fillet in the center of the foil, then season with lemon-pepper seasoning, drizzle with lemon juice, and top with 1 tablespoon butter.

Gently crimp the edges of foil to form a packet and place it into a 6-quart slow cooker.

Plugin the slow cooker, shut with lid, and cook for 3 hours at high heat or until cooked.

Serve straight away.

Nutrition:

Calories: 201.2

Fat: 12.9g

Protein: 19.6g

Carbs: 1.5g

Fiber: 0.3g

Sugar: 0.7g

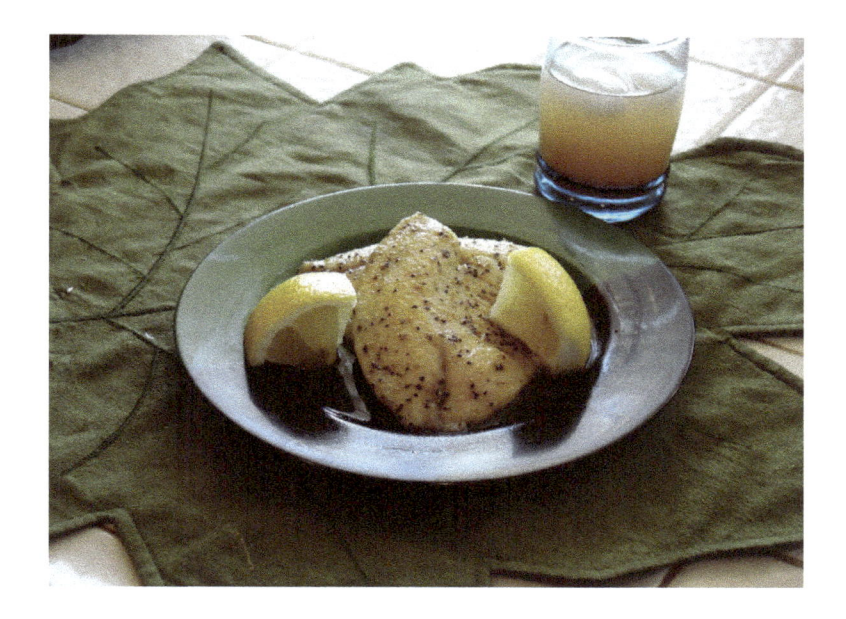

Poached Salmon in Court-Bouillon Recipe

Preparation Time: 5 minutes

Cooking Time: 2 hours 30 minutes

Servings: 2

Ingredients:

2 whole black peppercorns

1/2 medium carrot, thinly sliced

1/2 celery rib, thinly sliced

2 salmon steaks in 1-inch-thick slices

1 1/2 tbsp white wine vinegar

Directions:

Put all the items in the crockpot except for the salmon. You can also add parsley and bay leaf for extra flavor.

Rub salmon slices with salt and pepper to taste.

Cook within 2 hours on high.

Put some of the liquid over the top. Cook again within 30 minutes, high.

Nutrition:

Calories: 197

Fat: 7.7g

Carbs: 4.8g

Protein: 18.3g

Cholesterol: 95mg

Sodium: 366mg

Braised Squid with Tomatoes and Fennel

Preparation Time: 20 minutes

Cooking Time: 4 hours

Servings: 2

Ingredients:

1 1/2 cups clam juice

1 can plum tomatoes

1/2 fennel bulb, minced

3 tbsp all-purpose flour

1 lb. squid in 1-inch pieces

Directions:

Add chopped onions, fennel, and garlic to the flameproof insert of a crockpot and cook on a stove in medium heat for about 5 minutes.

Whisk in flour and tomato paste until thoroughly mixed, then add the clam juice, tomatoes, 1 tsp salt, and pepper. Boil for about 2 minutes.

Transfer to the crockpot, cover, and cook for 3 hours on low.

Uncover, add the squid and mix well—Cook for another 1 hour.

Nutrition:

Calories: 210

Fat: 25g

Carbs: 6g

Protein: 29g

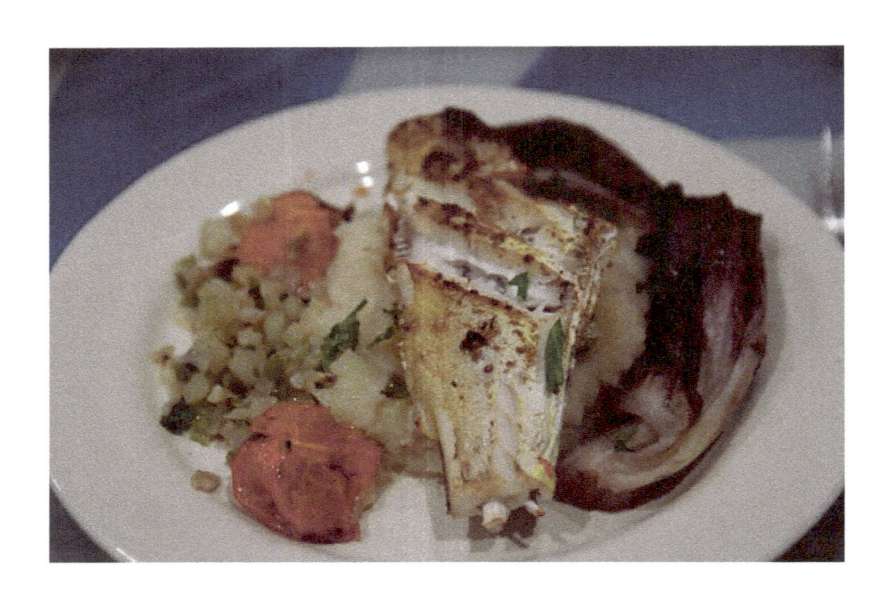

Seafood Stir-Fry Soup

Preparation Time: 30 minutes

Cooking Time: 3 hours & 10 minutes

Servings: 2

Ingredients:

7.25 oz low-carb Udon noodle, beef flavor

1/2 lb. shrimp

1/4 lb. scallops

3 cups low-sodium broth

1 carrot, shredded

Directions:

Add all ingredients except noodles, shrimp, and scallops to the crockpot. Include seasonings such as garlic, ginger, salt, and pepper to taste. Add vinegar, soy sauce, and fish sauce, 1/2 tbsp each. Stir to mix well.

Cook on high for 2-3 hours. Add udon noodles, shrimp, and scallops. Cook on high for additional 10-15 minutes.

Nutrition:

Calories: 266

Fat: 19g

Carbs: 8g

Protein: 27.5g

Cholesterol: 173mg

Sodium: 489mg

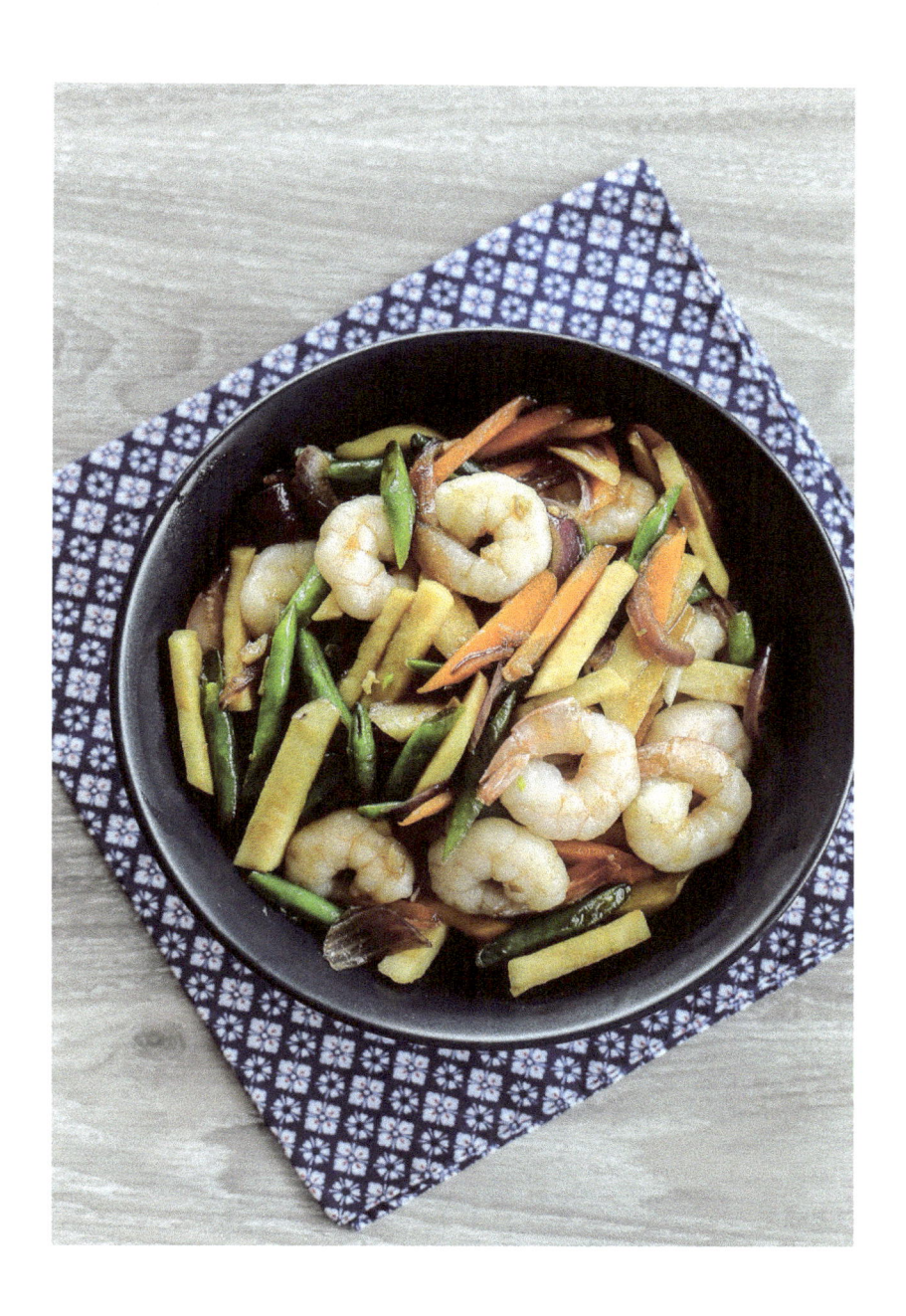

Shrimp Fajita Soup

Preparation Time: 20 minutes

Cooking Time: 2 hours

Servings: 2

Ingredients:

1/2 lb. shrimp

32 oz chicken broth

1 tbsp fajita seasoning

1/2 bell pepper, sliced or diced

Directions:

Put all the listed items except the shrimp in the crockpot. Add onion slices to taste and stir to mix well. Cook on high for 2 hours. Add the shrimp, and cook for additional 5-15 minutes.

Nutrition:

Calories: 165

Fat: 7.3g

Carbs: 3.7g

Protein: 15.9g

Cholesterol: 87mg

Sodium: 215mg

Fish and Tomatoes

Preparation Time: 7 minutes

Cooking Time: 3 hours

Servings: 2

Ingredients:

1/2 bell pepper, sliced

1/8 cup low-sodium broth

8 oz diced tomatoes

1/2 tbsp rosemary

1/2 lb. cod

Directions:

Put all the listed fixing except the fish in the crockpot. Add garlic, salt, and pepper to taste.

Season fish with your favorite seasoning and place other ingredients in the pot. Cook for 3 hours on low.

Nutrition:

Calories: 204

Fat: 16.8g

Carbs: 5g

Protein: 25.3g

Cholesterol: 75mg

Sodium: 296mg

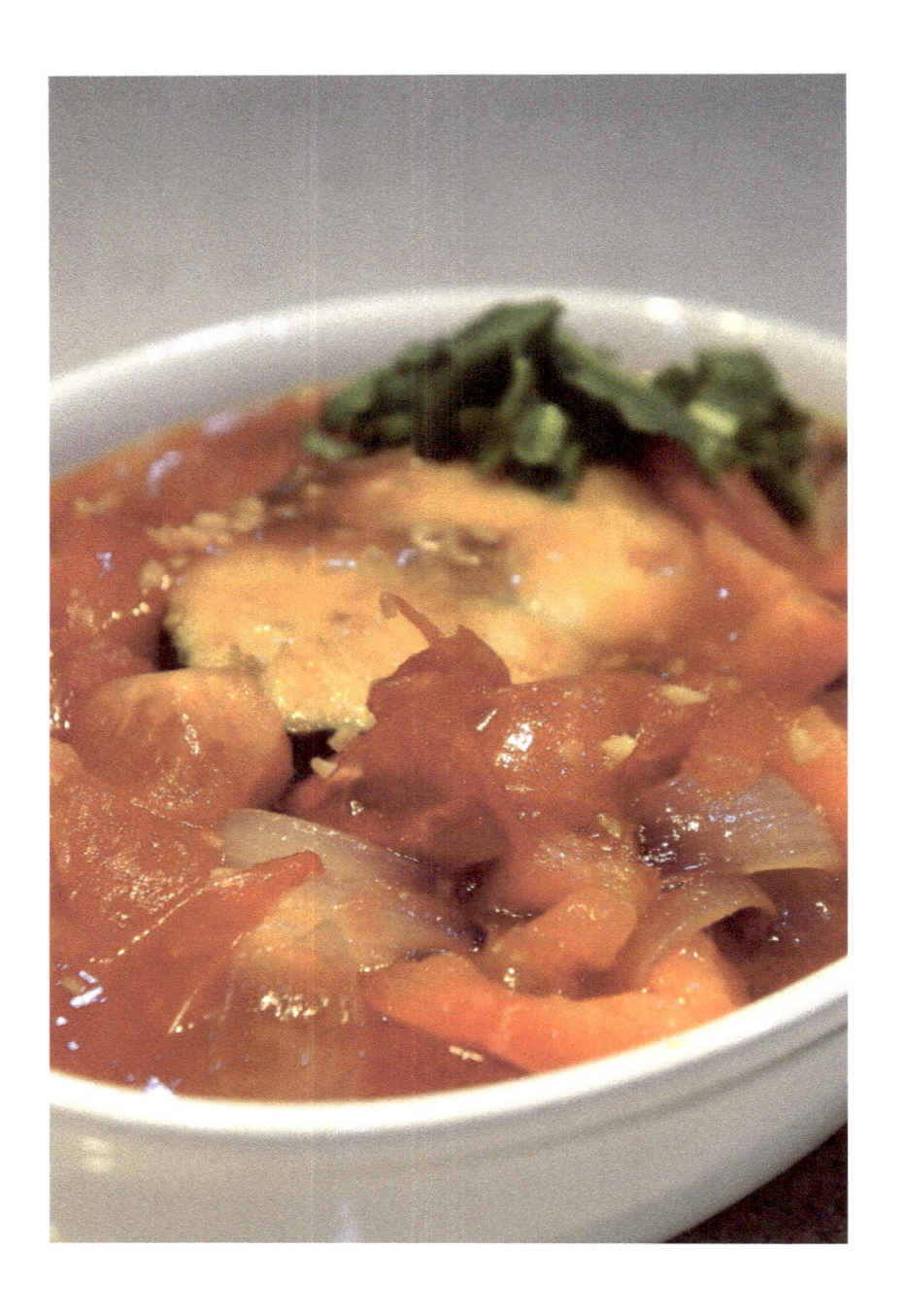

Vegetables

Parmesan Mushrooms

Preparation Time: 5 minutes

Cooking Time: 4 hours

Servings: 4

Ingredients:

16 oz. cremini mushrooms, fresh

½ oz. ranch dressing mix

2 tbsp. parmesan cheese, add more if desired

½ cup butter, melted and unsalted

Directions

Place the mushrooms in the slow cooker.

Combine melted butter and ranch dressing in a small-sized bowl. Stir in the butter mixture over the mushrooms and mix well.

Now, toss the parmesan cheese over the top. Cover the slow cooker and cook for 4 hours on low heat.

Nutrition:

Calories: 240

Carbs: 4g

Protein: 4.9g

Fat: 24g

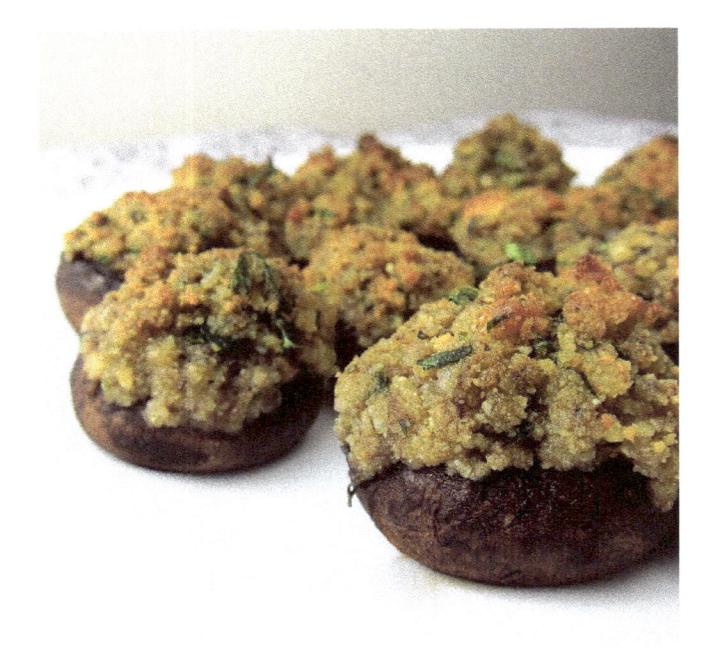

Mashed Garlic Cauliflower

Preparation Time: 5 minutes

Cooking Time: 6 hours

Servings: 6

Ingredients:

2 medium cauliflower head, sliced into florets

3 tbsp. butter

4 garlic cloves

2 tsp Celtic sea salt

8 to 10 cups of water

½ tsp black pepper

Dill, to taste

Directions:

Place the garlic and cauliflower along with a sufficient amount of water in the slow cooker.

Cook within 6 hours on low heat or until the cauliflower becomes tender.

Discard the water then place the cauliflower in the food processor. Add butter, then pulse until it is mashed.

Now, to this, stir in the seasoning and check for taste. Finally, toss the herbs into it and serve it immediately.

Nutrition:

Calories: 58

Carbs: 0.5g

Protein: 0.2g

Fat: 1.4g

Braised Cabbage

Preparation Time: 5 minutes

Cooking Time: 5 hours

Servings: 2

Ingredients:

1 green cabbage head, tough ends discarded and cut into 12 wedges

½ cup bone broth

1 sweet onion, preferably large and chopped

¼ cup bacon fat, melted

4 garlic cloves

Celtic sea salt, preferably coarse

caraway seeds

Directions:

Heat the slow cooker on high heat and then add melted bacon fat and onions to it.

After that, place the cabbage wedges in a layer in the slow cooker. Spoon the broth over it along with the salt and caraway seeds.

Cover the slow cooker, then cook within 1 hour. In between, stir the cabbage once to shift the top ones to the bottom. Pour in more stock if required.

Cook it again for another 4 hours on high heat. Once cooked, you can add some apple cider vinegar if you like.

Nutrition:

Calories: 122

Carbs: 2g

Protein: 8.7g

Fat: 3.4g

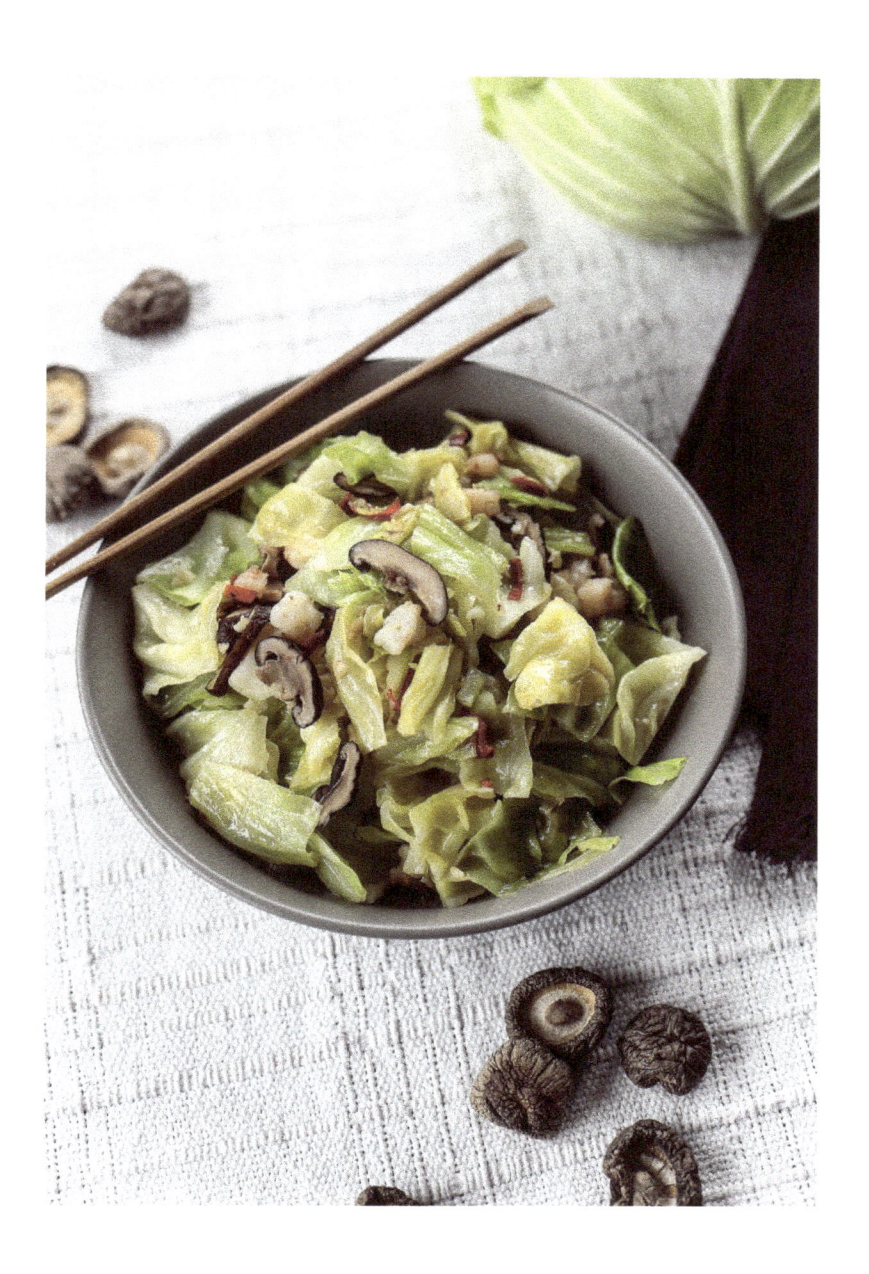

Homemade Vegetable Stock

Preparation Time: 15 minutes

Cooking Time: 12 hours & 30 minutes

Servings: 4

Ingredients:

4 quarts cold filtered water

12 whole peppercorns

3 peeled and chopped carrots

3 chopped celery stalks

2 bay leaves

4 smashed garlic cloves

1 large quartered onion

2 tablespoons apple cider vinegar

Any other vegetable scraps

Directions:

Put everything in your slow cooker and cover. Do not turn on; let it sit for 30 minutes.

Cook on low for 12 hours. Strain the broth and discard the solids.

Before using, keep the stock in a container in the fridge for 2-3 hours.

Nutrition:

Calories: 11

Protein: 0g

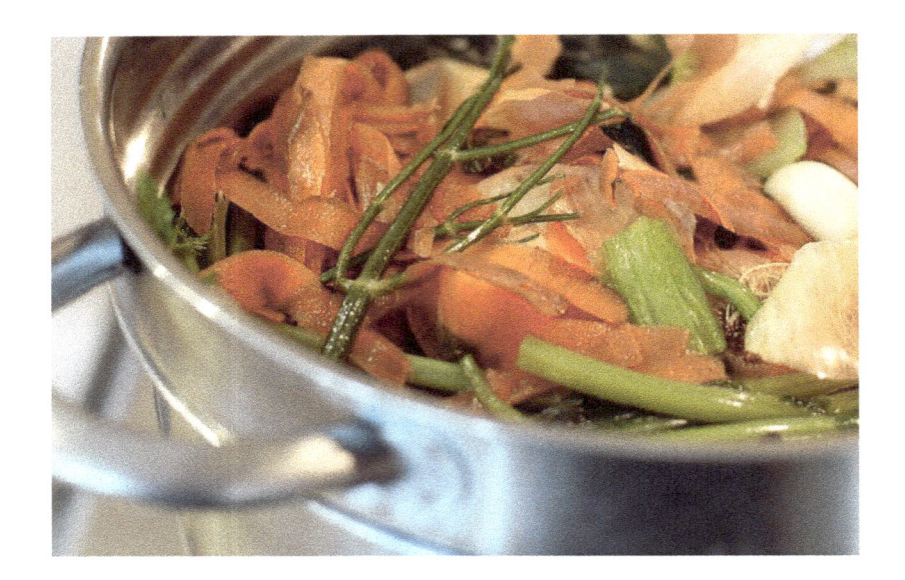

Carbs: 3g
Fat: 0g
Fiber: 0g

Vegetable Korma

Preparation Time: 15 minutes

Cooking Time: 8 hours

Servings: 4

Ingredients:

1 head's worth of cauliflower florets

¾ can of full-fat coconut milk

2 cups chopped green beans

½ chopped onion

2 minced garlic cloves

2 tablespoons curry powder

2 tablespoons coconut flour

1 teaspoon garam masala

Salt and pepper to taste

Directions:

Add vegetables into your slow cooker. Mix coconut milk with seasonings.

Pour into the slow cooker. Sprinkle over coconut flour and mix until blended.

Close and cook on low for 8 hours. Taste and season more if necessary. Serve!

Nutrition:
Calories: 206
Protein: 5g
Carbs: 18g
Fat: 14g
Fiber: 9.5g

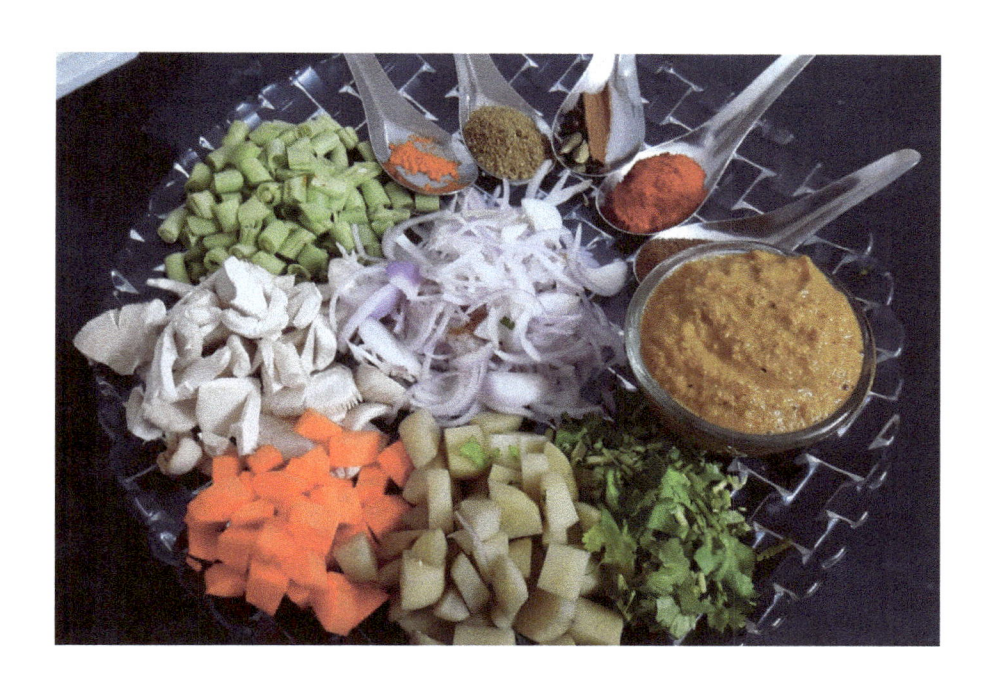

Stuffed Eggplant

Preparation Time: 15 minutes

Cooking Time: 1 hour & 30 minutes

Servings: 6

Ingredients:

1 seeded and chopped green bell pepper

1 tbsp. tomato paste

1 tsp. cumin

1 tsp. raw coconut sugar

2 chopped red onions

3 tbsp. chopped parsley

4 chopped tomatoes

4 minced garlic cloves

4 tbsp. olive oil

6 eggplants

Directions:

Remove eggplant skins with a vegetable peeler. Slice eggplants lengthwise and sprinkle with salt. Set aside for half an hour to sweat.

Place eggplants into your slow cooker. Cook on high 20 minutes.

Sauté onions in a heated pan with olive oil. Stir bell pepper and garlic with onions and sauté for an additional 1 to 2 minutes.

Pour mixture into eggplants into the slow cooker—Cook 20 minutes on high.

Put pepper plus salt and add parsley, tomato paste, cumin, sugar, and tomato. Cook another 10 minutes, stir well and serve!

Nutrition:

Calories: 180

Carbs: 2g

Fat: 13g

Protein: 9g

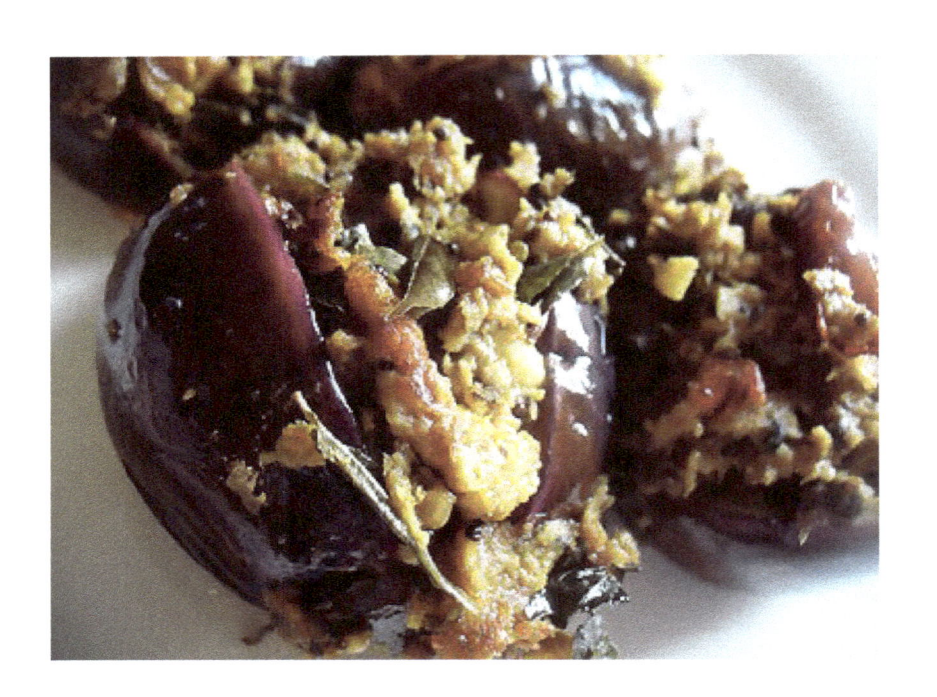

Bacon Cheddar Broccoli Salad

Preparation Time: 15 minutes

Cooking Time: 2 hours

Servings: 15

Ingredients:

Dressing:

¼ C. sweetener of choice

1 C. keto mayo

2 tbsp. organic vinegar

Broccoli Salad:

½ diced red onion

4 ounces cheddar cheese

½ pound bacon, cooked and chopped

1 large head broccoli

1/8 C. sunflower seeds

1/8 C. pumpkin seeds

Directions:

For the dressing, whisk all dressing components together, adjusting taste pepper and salt, and add to your slow cooker. Set to a low setting to cook for 2 hours until everything is combined. Serve warm!

Nutrition:

Calories: 189

Carbs: 8g

Fat: 21g
Protein: 8g

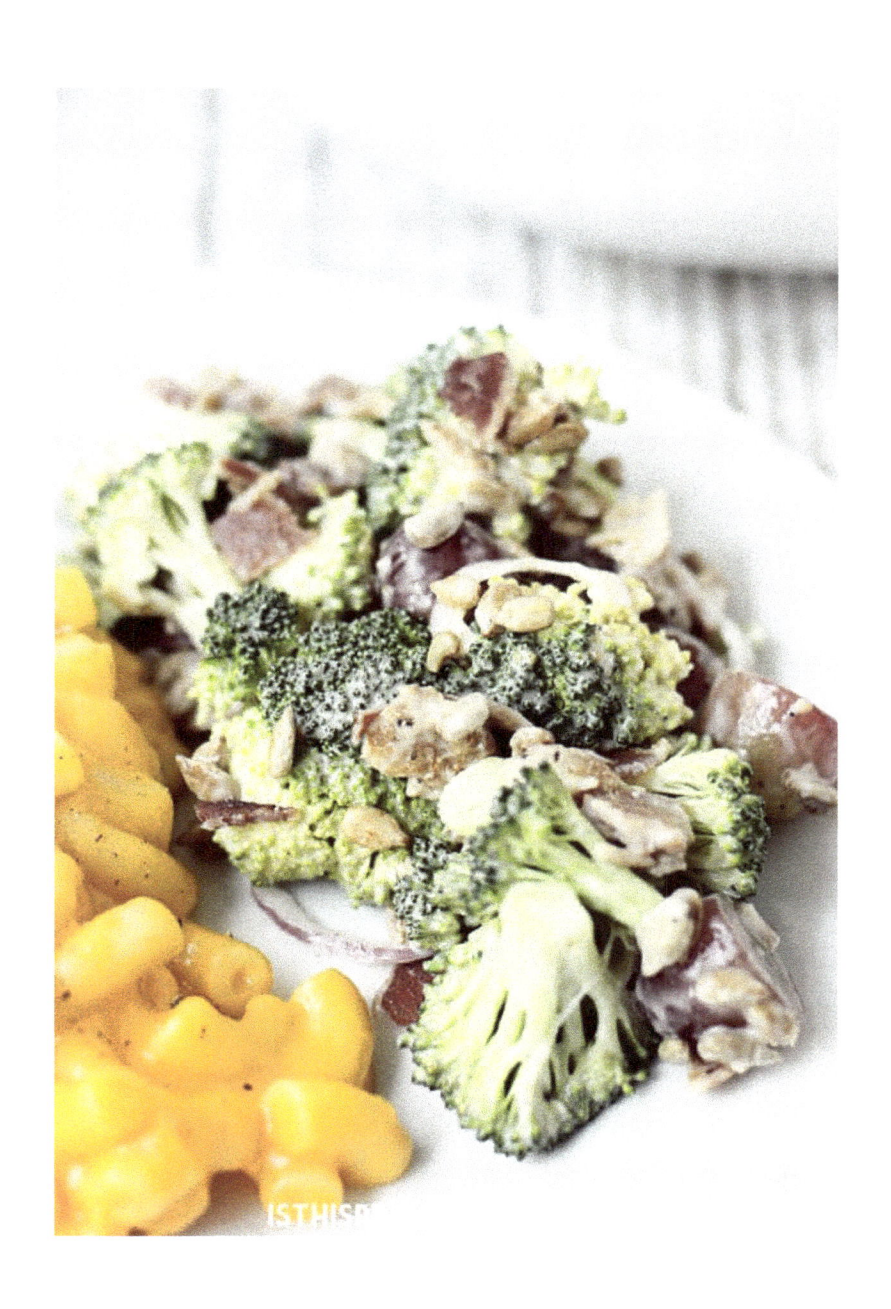

Cracked-Out Keto Slaw

Preparation Time: 15 minutes

Cooking Time: 1 hour & 35 minutes

Servings: 2

Ingredients:

½ C. chopped macadamia nuts

1 tbsp. sesame oil

1 tsp. chili paste

1 tsp. vinegar

2 garlic cloves

2 tbsp. tamari

4 C. shredded cabbage

Directions:

Toss cabbage with chili paste, sesame oil, vinegar, and tamari. Add to slow cooker.

Add minced garlic and mix well. Set to cook on high 1 ½ hours.

Stir in macadamia nuts. Cook 5 minutes more.

Garnish with sesame seeds before serving.

Nutrition:

Calories: 360

Carbs: 5g

Fat: 33g

Protein: 7g

Zucchini Pasta

Preparation Time: 15 minutes

Cooking Time: 2 hours

Servings: 4

Ingredients:

¼ C. olive oil

½ C. basil

½ tsp. red pepper flakes

1-pint halved cherry tomatoes

1 sliced red onion

2 pounds spiralized zucchini

4 minced garlic cloves

Directions:

Sauté onion and garlic 3 minutes till fragrant in olive oil.

Add zucchini noodles to your slow cooker and season with pepper and salt—Cook 60 minutes on high heat. Mix in tomatoes, basil, onion, garlic, and red pepper. Cook another 20 minutes.

Add parmesan cheese to slow cooker. Mix thoroughly and cook 10 minutes to melt the cheese. Devour!

Nutrition:

Calories: 181

Carbs: 6g

Fat: 13g
Protein: 5g

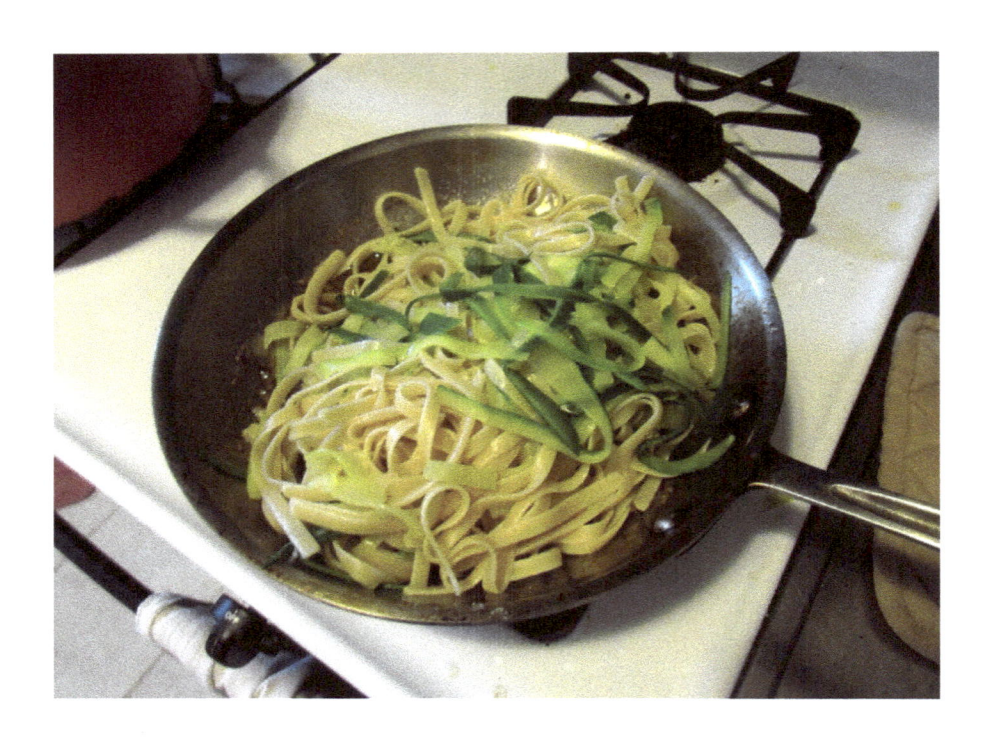

Twice Baked Spaghetti Squash

Preparation Time: 15 minutes

Cooking Time: 6 hours

Servings: 4

Ingredients:

¼ tsp. Pepper

¼ tsp. salt

½ C. grated parmesan cheese

1 tsp. oregano

2 minced garlic cloves

2 small spaghetti squashes

2 tbsp. butter

4 slices Provolone cheese

Directions:

Cut spaghetti squash in half lengthwise, discarding innards. Set gently into your pot.

Cook on high heat for 4 hours.

Take squash innards and mix with parmesan cheese and butter. Then mix in pepper, salt, garlic, and oregano.

Add squash innards mixture to the middle of cooked squash halves.

Cook on high for another 1-2 hours till middles are deliciously bubbly.

Nutrition:

Calories: 230

Carbs: 4g

Fat: 17g

Protein: 12g

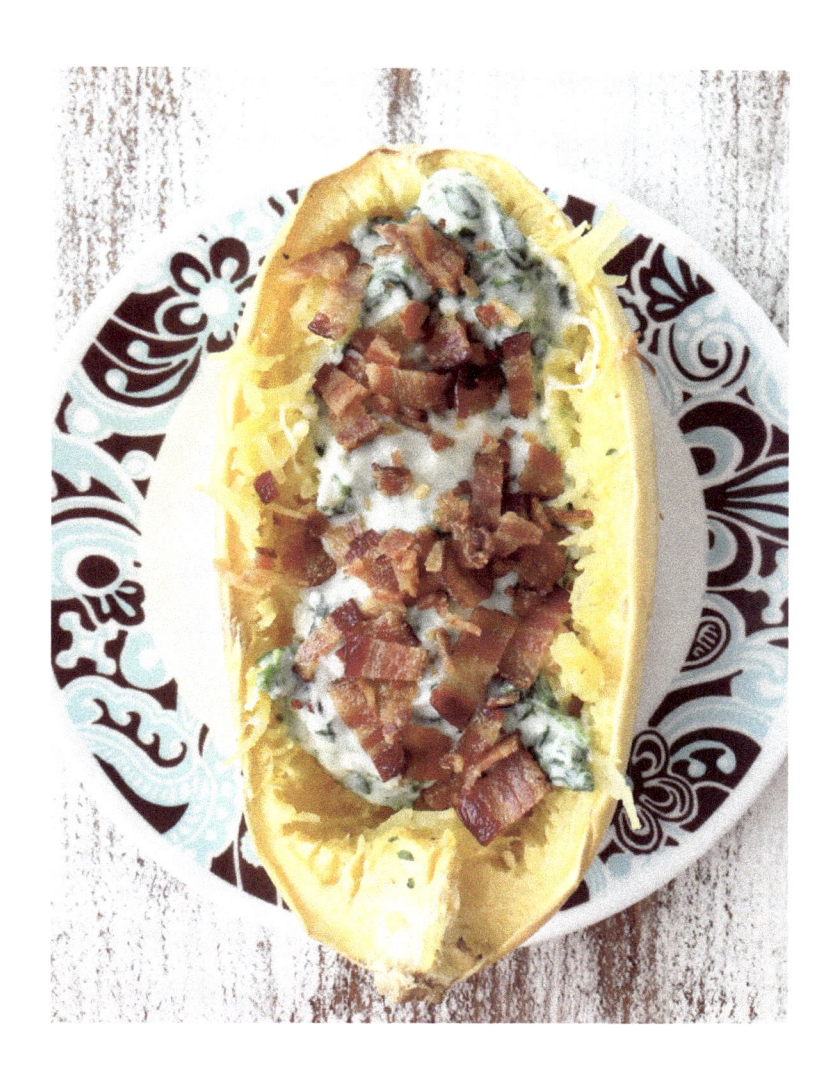

Mushroom Risotto

Preparation Time: 15 minutes

Cooking Time: 4 hours

Servings: 4

Ingredients:

¼ C. vegetable broth

1-pound sliced Portobello mushrooms

1-pound sliced white mushrooms

1/3 C. grated parmesan cheese

2 diced shallots

3 tbsp. chopped chives

3 tbsp. coconut oil

4 ½ C. riced cauliflower

4 tbsp. butter

Directions:

Heat-up oil and sauté mushrooms 3 minutes till soft. Discard liquid and set it to the side.

Add oil to skillet and sauté shallots 60 seconds.

Pour all recipe components into your pot and mix well to combine.

Cook 3 hours on high heat. Serve topped with parmesan cheese.

Nutrition:

Calories: 438

Carbs: 5g

Fat: 17g

Protein: 12g

Vegan Bibimbap

Preparation Time: 15 minutes

Cooking Time: 45 minutes

Servings: 4

Ingredients:

½ cucumber, sliced into strips

1 grated carrot

1 sliced red bell pepper

1 tbsp. soy sauce

1 tsp. sesame oil

10-ounces riced cauliflower

2 tbsp. rice vinegar

2 tbsp. sesame seeds

2 tbsp. sriracha sauce

4-5 broccoli florets

7-ounces tempeh, sliced into squares

Liquid sweetener

Directions:

In a bowl, combine tempeh squares with 1 tbsp soy sauce and 2 tbsp vinegar. Set aside to soak. Slice veggies.

Add carrot, broccoli, and peppers to slow cooker. Cook on high 30 minutes.

Add cauliflower rice to the slow cooker; cook 5 minutes.

Add sweetener, oil, soy sauce, vinegar, and sriracha to slow cooker. Don't hesitate to add a bit of water if you find the mixture to be too thick.

Nutrition:

Calories: 119

Carbs: 0g

Fat: 18g

Protein: 8g

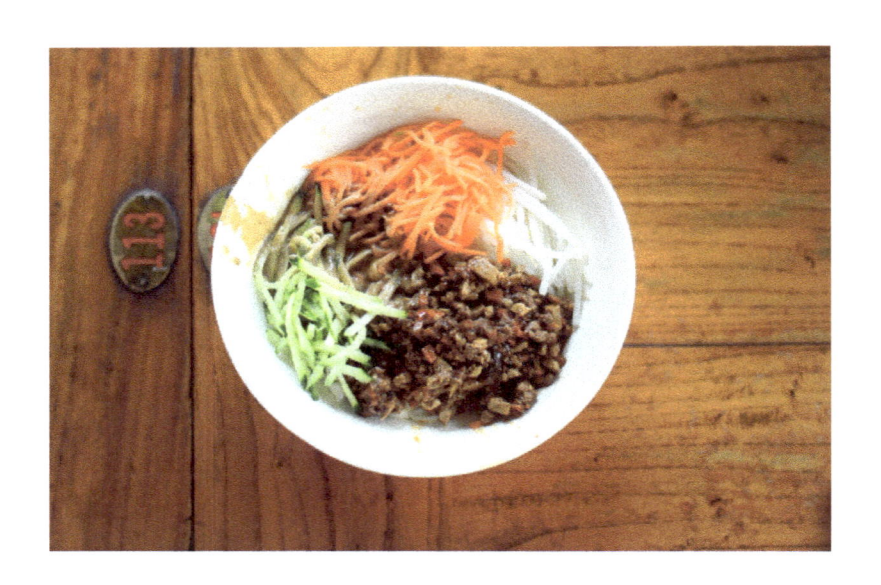

Avocado Pesto Kelp Noodles

Preparation Time: 15 minutes

Cooking Time: 1 hour & 30 minutes

Servings: 2

Ingredients:

Pesto:

¼ C. basil

½ C. extra-virgin olive oil

1 avocado

1 C. baby spinach leaves

1 tsp. salt

1-2 garlic cloves

1 package of kelp noodles

Directions:

Add kelp noodles to slow cooker with just enough water to cover them. Cook on high 45-60 minutes. In the meantime, combine pesto ingredients in a blender, blending till smooth and incorporated. Stir in pesto and heat noodle mixture 10 minutes.

Nutrition:

Calories: 321

Carbs: 1g

Fat: 32g

Protein: 2g

pinkwhen

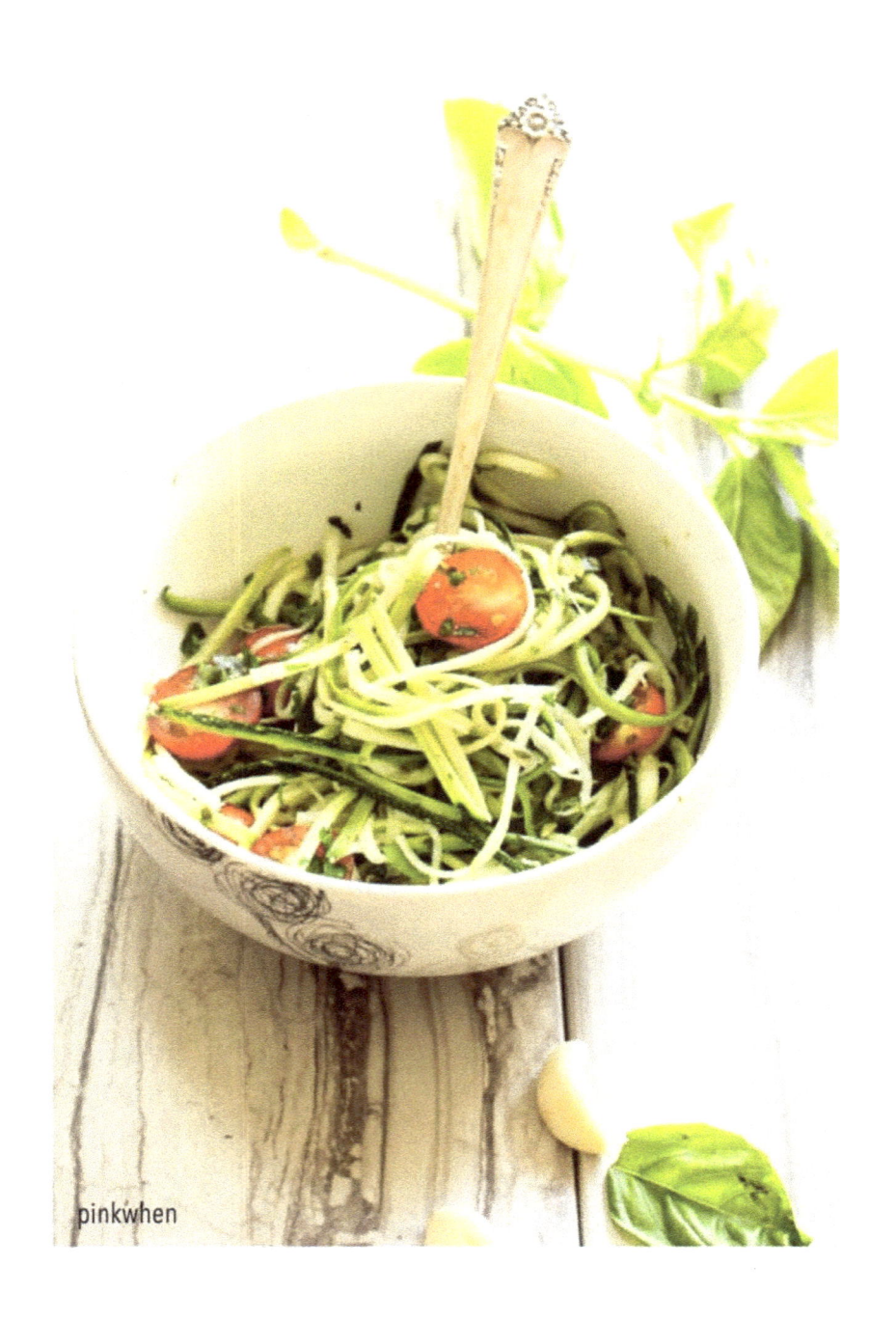

Creamy Curry Sauce Noodle Bowl

Preparation Time: 15 minutes

Cooking Time: 2 hours

Servings: 4

Ingredients:

½ head chopped cauliflower

1 diced red bell pepper

1 pack of Kanten Noodles

2 chopped carrots

2 handfuls of mixed greens

Chopped cilantro

Curry Sauce:

¼ C. avocado oil mayo

¼ C. water

¼ tsp./ ginger

½ tsp. pepper

1 ½ tsp. coriander

1 tsp. cumin

1 tsp turmeric

2 tbsp. apple cider vinegar

2 tbsp. avocado oil

2 tsp. curry powder

Directions:

Add all ingredients, minus curry sauce components, to your slow cooker. Set to cook on high 1-2 hours.

In the meantime, add all of the curry sauce ingredients to a blender. Puree until smooth.

Pour over veggie and noodle mixture. Stir well to coat.

Nutrition:

Calories: 110

Carbs: 1g

Fat: 9g

Protein: 7g

Lightning Source UK Ltd.
Milton Keynes UK
UKHW021852130121
376954UK00001B/19